Health

The Vocabulary of Our Bodies and Health Care

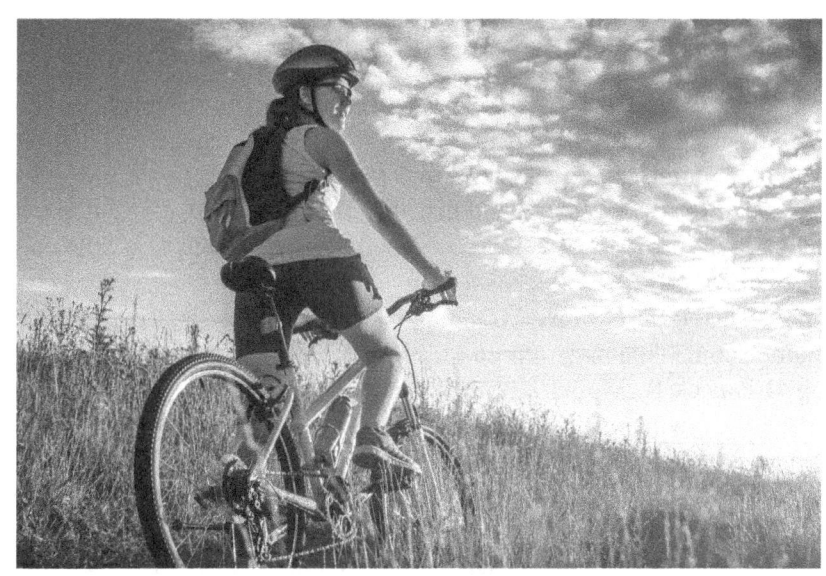

Raymond C. Clark

PRO LINGUA
LEARNING

Pro Lingua Learning
PO Box 4467
Rockville, MD 20849
Office: 1-301-424-8900
Book orders: 1-800-888-4741
Web: ProLinguaLearning.com
Email: Info@ProLinguaLearning.com

***At Pro Lingua**
our objective is to foster an approach
to learning and teaching that we call
interplay, the **inter**action of language
learners and teachers with their materials,
with the language and culture,
and with each other in active, creative,
and productive **play**.*

Health: Vocabulary of Our Bodies and Health Care was designed and set in Adobe Times New Roman by Arthur A. Burrows. This is a digital font based on an early twentieth-century old-fashioned serif type called Times New Roman, commissioned by the British newspaper *The Times* in 1931 and designed by Victor Lardent for the Monotype company. Digitized and distributed with Microsoft products, it has become one of the most widely used typefaces in history. It is easy to read, with strong contrasting bold and italic faces.

The front cover photo is 76390914 © Rawpixelimages | Dreamstime.com. Back cover photo is 76786358 © Ammentorp | Dreamstime.com. Title page: Photo 113753628 / Healthy Lifestyle © Mariia Boiko | Dreamstime. com. Page 1 drawing © Patrick R. Moran/*Lexicarry*. Page 5 Photo 30079295 Skeleton © Alexander Potapov | Dreamstime.com. Page 9 drawings © Patrick R. Moran/*Faces*. Page 13 Photo 43101986 Earache © Renaud Philippe | Dreamstime.com. Page 17 Digestive tract © NIH. Page 21 Blood Drive image No, 11© American Red Cross. Page 32 Photo 33264519 filling outform © Robert Kneschke | Dreamstime.com. Page 33 *Nasreddin Hodja* © Raymond C. Clark/ Robert MacLean. Page 37 Photo 1951204 hospital © Tom Fawls | Dreamstime.com. Page 41 vegetables ID 1430407 © Og-vision | Dreamstime.com; fruit Photo 2999796 © Andrey Armyagov | Dreamstime.com. Page 45 gym Photo 79791734 © Mirko Vitali | Dreamstime.com; treadmill Photo 120293349 © Mladen Zivkovic | Dreamstime.com. Page 53 Photo facemask79791734 © Mirko Vitali |Dreamstime.com. Page 57 birth Photo 79791734 © Mirko Vitali | Dreamstime.com; hospice Photo 63171166 © Katarzyna Bialasiewicz | Dreamstime.com. Page 60 Photo 96927265 © Msalena | Dreamstime.com Shakespeare with a skull in Madame Tussaud`s museum. Berlin, Germany.

Contents: Health Lessons with Vocabulary

Thanks

Many thanks to my daughter Susannah Clark, PA for her review of my first, very rough attempt to write about the basics of health care, and for her second look at my improvements.

For the last 40 + years I have written and co-written, and edited dozens of Pro Lingua Associates publications. We are now about to merge with Language Arts Press and become a new version of our labor of love, and this work is the last that was done with the support and assistance of my associates. First and foremost, Andy and Elise Burrows have been the mainstays of our company and the first people I have turned to as my work took shape and I needed commentary. Their response has been invaluable. And I should offer special mention to Andy, who has taken my rough drafts and made them into real books. And through the years I have always had the good fortune of exploring our profession and publications with our associates, Pat Moran and Mike Jerald. That association will continue, and we look forward to a new professional association with Michael Berman of Language Arts Press.

RCC

Introduction and User's Guide

The purpose of this book is to help English language learners increase their vocabulary in the semantic field of health. A secondary purpose is to increase awareness of and knowledge about personal and public health, an important aspect of everyone's everyday life.

The individual units are photocopyable so that users may select material that is appropriate. Copying the entire book is not permitted.

Health is appropriate for intermediate English language learners from middle school to adult. It would also be suitable for native speakers who need to improve their vocabulary in the area of health care. It can be used by individuals in a class setting or by individuals doing self-study. The audio component could be especially helpful for the self-studier.

There are 15 units. The units proceed from easiest and shortest to more difficult. It is recommended that you begin with *Unit One, The Body* and proceed unit by unit to the last unit, *Birth and Death*. A lot of the vocabulary and concepts naturally recycle. For example, the parts of the body in Unit One will recur in subsequent units.

The units follow a four-page format. Each unit also has an audio component that includes the main reading passage of the unit and the applications. The use of the audio is optional, but it can help the learners' listening comprehension and pronunciation.

PAGE 1. **Awareness Openers.** The first page of the unit introduces the subject. It is intended to be an attention-getting prompt promoting awareness of the topic. There is no single, simple way to use this page; the objective is to have the learner begin to think about the topic. A simple way to get started is for pairs or small groups prompted by the teacher to talk to each other about the page. The first page also lists the key words that will be found on the next page. One way to use this list is to have the learners first talk about and explain the familiar words to each other and then guess the new words. This will help with the comprehension of the following page.

PAGE 2. **The Reading.** This is the heart of the unit – a reading/listening passage. Key words are highlighted in the reading. In most cases, the context will help the learner understand the meaning of the key words. The reading may be used in a number of ways, but a simple and effective way is for the teacher to read the passage aloud while the learners simply listen. An alternative is to play the audio. Then the learners read the passage silently as individuals. When all have finished, the teacher asks for questions or asks questions. Not everyone will finish at the same time, so early finishers can be encouraged to go on to the exercises.

PAGE 3. **Exercises**. These two exercises are a comprehension check and a "second look" at the passage, exploring the form, meaning, and usage of the key words. The answers are in the back of the book.

For the Matching Exercise the learners will need to consider syntax as well as the meaning of the sentence as they search for the match. In other words, the learners will also be activating their use of the grammar.

The exercises can be done by independent learners or in class by individuals or by pairs working together.

PAGE 4. **Applications.** This page has a variety of activities intended to explore the topic of the unit. It also asks the learners to be creative and think critically.

There is a key word index in the back of the book that lists and locates the first occurrence of each lexical item. The numbers indicate the Unit. There are 205 items.

1. The Body

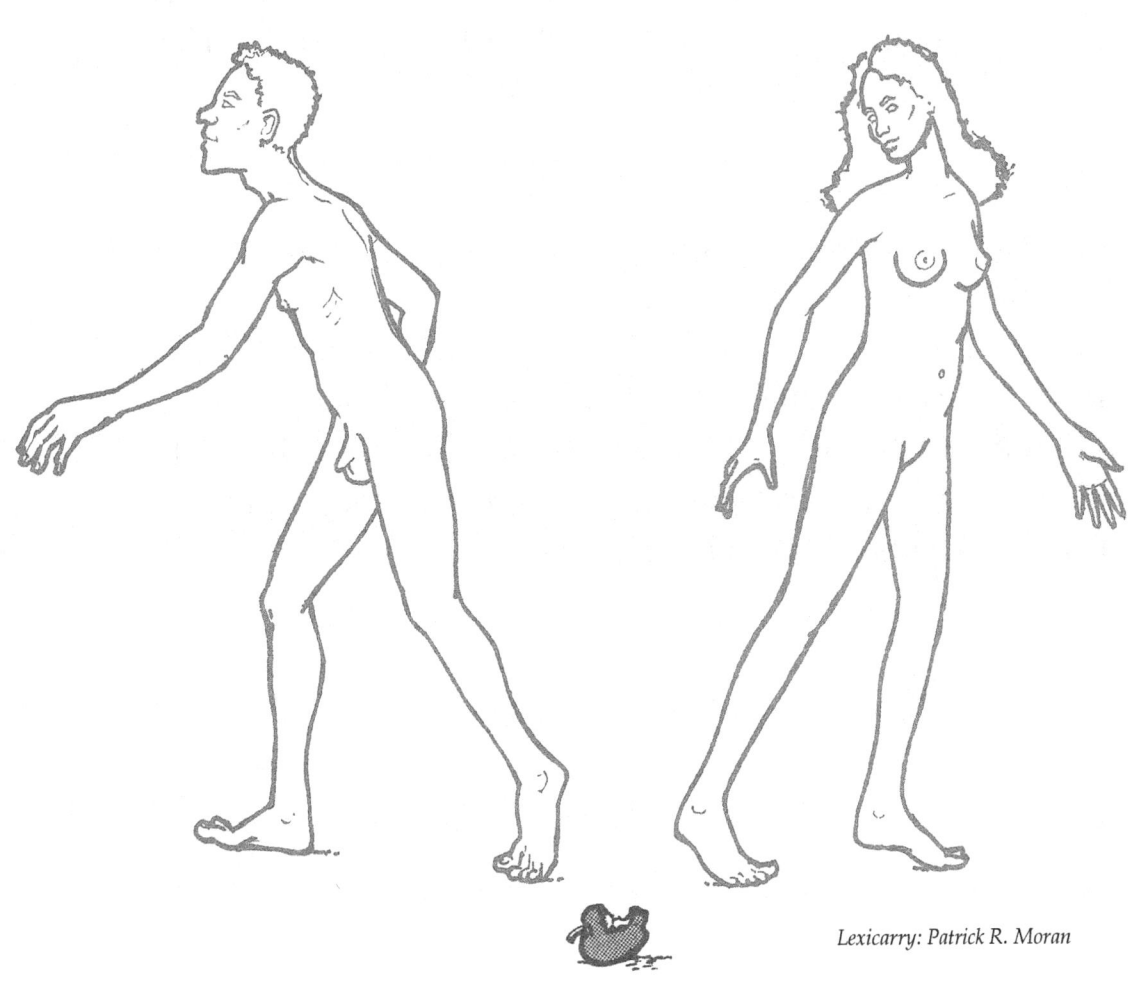

Lexicarry: Patrick R. Moran

Key Words

male	female	arm	leg
hand	finger	foot/feet	toe
head	stomach	chest	breast
hair			

The **male** body and the **female** body are different; they are also the same in many ways. They both have two **arms** and two **legs**. Their arms have **hands** and their hands have **fingers**. Their legs have **feet** and their feet have **toes**. They have a **head**, but their heads are a little different.

The main part of the human body has the **stomach** and the **chest** on the front side, and the **back** is on the other side. The female chest has **breast**s.

Both males and females have **hair** on their heads. Men often have hair on their faces, stomachs, and chests. Both men and women have hair on their arms and legs, but usually men have more hair. *(120)*

EXERCISES
(*answers on page 61*)

A. Match the two parts of the sentence.

1. The chest is not _____	A. toes.
2. Another word for men_____	B. hair on his legs.
3. The stomach _____	C. on the back.
4. Their bodies are different, _____	D. on their heads.
5. Men often have _____	E. breasts on her chest.
6. The feet have ten _____	F. have fingers.
7. They have hair_____	G. hair on their chests.
8. A woman has _____	H. but also the same.
9. A man has more _____	I. is males.
10. Women are _____	J. is on the front of the body.
11. The hands_____	K. female.

B. Fill in each blank with the best word.

1. The stomach area is on the front and the _____ is on the other side.
2. Usually men have more _____ .
3. A woman's _____ has _____ .
4. The arms have _____ .
5. The _____ have feet.
6. A man is a _____ and a woman is a _____ .
7. A man is _____ and a woman is _____ .
8. We have ten _____ and ten _____ on our hands and feet.

THINK ABOUT IT
(What is the meaning of the underlined words?)

1. A: When I said I could do it, I really <u>put my foot in my mouth</u>.
   B: You don't know how to do it, do you?

2. A: I want to <u>get something off my chest</u>.
   B: Go ahead.
   A: What you said was really stupid.

3. A: What a storm!
   B: Yeah, the thunder and lightning was <u>hair-raising</u>.

4. A. Believe it or not, I won!
   B. I've got to <u>hand it to you</u>. I didn't think you could.

5. A: Please do this for me. I can't wait any longer.
   B: Okay, okay, stop <u>twisting my arm</u>, I'll do it.

6. A: This hotel seems a little expensive.
   B: It's okay. The company is <u>footing the bill</u>, not us.

7. A: This project will take some time.
   B: That's why I want to start now and <u>get a leg up on it.</u>

8. A: Come on. I know you've got my car keys. <u>Hand them over</u>.
   B: Here you are.

9. A: It looks pretty clear to me. It was his fault.
   B: You're right. He hasn't got <u>a leg to stand on</u> if it goes to court.

10. A: I told him to be careful. But he wasn't.
    B: He got into trouble, <u>lost his head</u>, and then did everything wrong.

2. The Skeleton

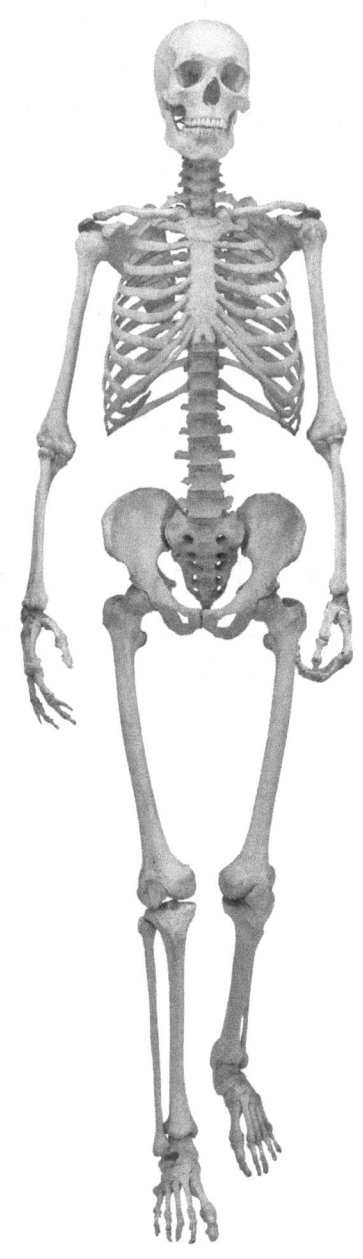

Key Words

skull	jaw	neck	vertebrae
spine	shoulder	elbow	wrist
hip	pelvis	thigh	knee
shin	ankle		

READ

Our body has a skeleton. It has 206 bones. This collection of bones lets us stand and move. The bone that is our head is the **skull**. It protects our brain. The skull has a moveable **jaw**. It lets us eat and speak. Our head is connected to the rest of our body by the **neck**. The neck bone is seven bones called **vertebrae**. The neck bones are the top part of the long backbone, or **spine**.

At the upper part of the body is the **shoulder**, a collection of bones that connect with the arm. The arm bends at a place called the **elbow,** and it also bends at the **wrist**, where it connects with our hand and its fingers.

At the **hip** area of our lower body is the **pelvis**. It connects with the legs. The upper leg bone, the **thigh** bone, connects to the lower leg at the **knee**. Below the knee there are two bones. The front one is the **shin**. At the base of the shin, the **ankle** connects to the foot with its toes.

The next time you stand up or sit down, think of how your skeleton is working together – a miracle in motion! *(201)*

EXERCISES
(answers on page 61)

A. Match the two parts of the sentence.

1. The neck bones _____   A. can move.
2. There are 206 bones _____   B. connects with the arm bone.
3. The spine _____   C. in the hip area.
4. The jaw _____   D. meet at the knee.
5. The shoulder _____   E. are called vertebrae.
6. The pelvis is _____   F. connect to the foot and hand.
7. The upper leg bone is_____   G. in the skeleton.
8. The thigh and shin _____   H. is the backbone.
9. The ankle and wrist _____   I. the thigh bone.

B. Fill in the blanks.

1. The bone that forms our head is the _____.
2. The _____ is moveable.
3. The _____ connects to the hand.
4. We bend the arm at the _____.
5. The _____ is in the hip area.
6. The _____ is between the foot and _____.
7. There are seven bones in the _____.
8. The leg bends at the _____.

THINK ABOUT IT

(What is the meaning of the underlined words?)

1. A: Oh, no! He threw the ball away!
    B: What a <u>bonehead</u> play!
    A: That <u>numbskull</u> should not be on the team.

2. A: Your father is professor of American history. Right?
    B: He is. And he loves to talk about it.
    A: I guess I better <u>bone up on</u> my history before we meet.

3. A: What weather! Have you been out to the lake?
    B: I have. It's <u>bone dry.</u>

4. A: He was lost in the desert for days.
    B: He was just <u>skin and bones</u> when they found him.

5. A: It seems the senator had <u>a skeleton in her closet</u>.
    B: Because of that, I think she will lose the election.

6. A: I've got <u>a bone to pick with you</u>. You told Maria I didn't like her hair style. Why did you say that?
    B: Sorry. My bad.

3. The Face

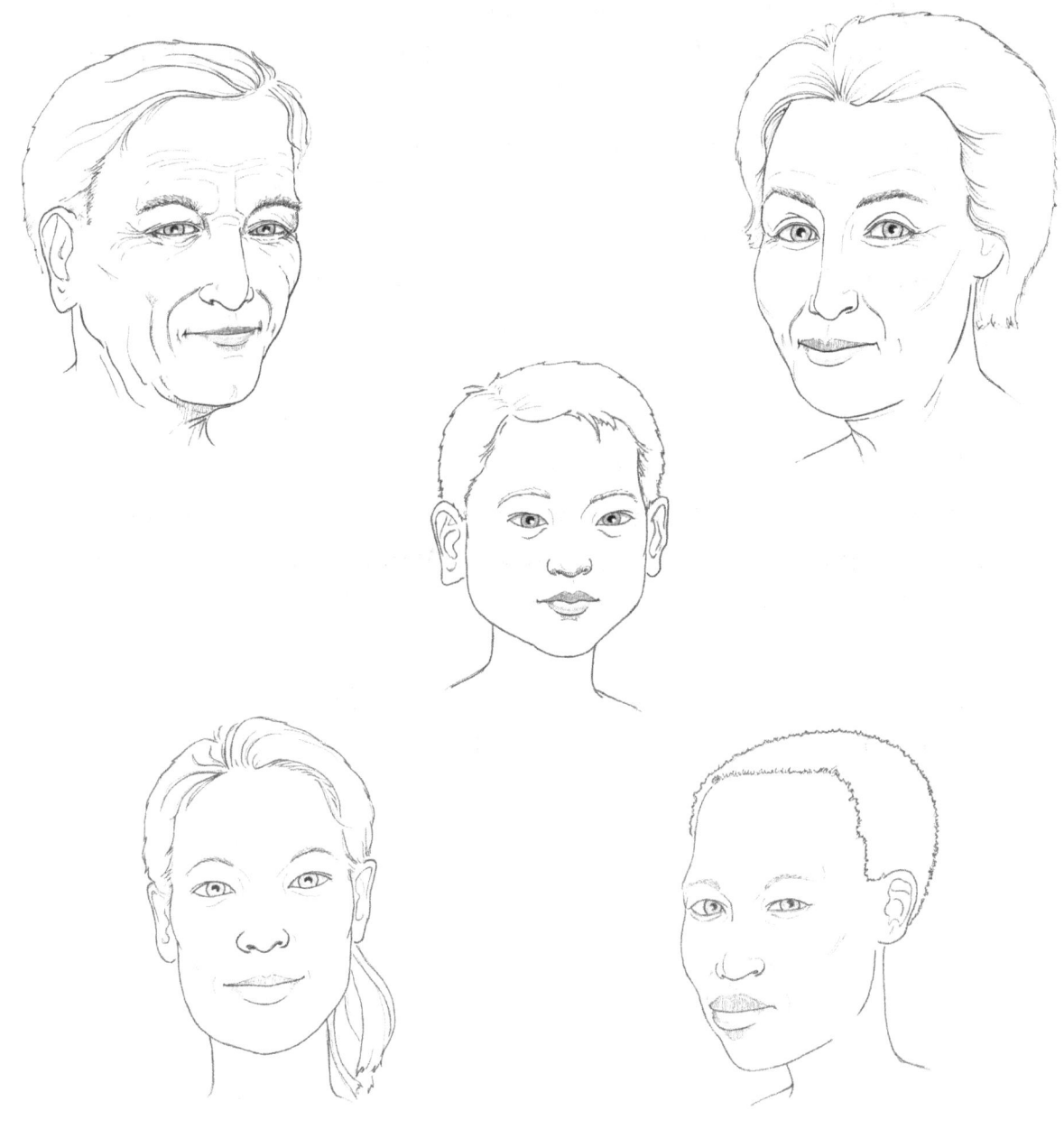

Faces: Patrick R. Moran

Key Words

eye	nose	mouth	to smell
to taste	eyelid	eyelash	eyebrow
lip	forehead	cheek	chin

Every person has a different **face**, but people everywhere have the same face. They have two **eyes**, one **nose**, and one **mouth**. They see with their eyes, **smell** with their nose, and **taste** with their mouth. The eyes have different colors; the most common color is brown. Other common colors are blue, green, and hazel. The eyes can be closed by closing the **eyelids**. The eyes have **eyelashes** on the lids of the eyes. The place above the eyes is the brow, and the hair on the brow is the **eyebrow**.

The nose is in the middle of the face. People's noses have different shapes. Some are long. Some are wide. Below the nose is the mouth. The **lips** are the outside part of the mouth. There are two lips – upper and lower. Mouths open and close. When the mouth is closed the lips touch each other.

The upper part of the face is the **forehead**. The sides of the face are the **cheeks**. The bottom of the face is the **chin**. *(172)*

EXERCISES
(answers on page 61)

A. Match the two parts of the sentence.

1. Every person _____	A. can close the eyes.
2. We smell _____	B. is the eyebrow.
3. The mouth has_____	C. and one chin.
4. Eyelids _____	D. on the eyelids.
5. The hair on the brow_____	E. has a different face.
6. The forehead_____	F. with our mouth.
7. We have two cheeks_____	G. different shapes.
8. Eyelashes are _____	H. with our nose.
9. Noses have _____	I. is the upper part of the face.
10. We taste _____	J. two lips.

B. Fill in the blanks.

1. My _____ are hazel.
2. The _____ is at the bottom of the face.
3. The nose is between the _____ and the eyes.
4. The _____ are part of the mouth.
5. Eye colors are hazel, blue, green, and _____.
6. We close our eyes with our _____.
7. _____ are actually hair.
8. The _____ is above the eyes and the eyebrows.
9. My _____ are on both sides of my nose.
10. We _____ with our noses and _____ with our mouths.

THINK ABOUT IT
(What is the meaning of the underlined words?)

1. A: Let's <u>face it,</u> we won't get there on time.
   B: Yeah, the plane leaves in ten minutes.

2. A: Can we meet on Zoom?
   B: I really prefer <u>face-to-face.</u>

3. A: Please don't tell anyone about this.
   B: My <u>lips are sealed</u>.

4. A: That politician is a <u>two-faced</u> liar.
   B: He says one thing and does another.

5. A: My neighbor watches everything I do. I don't like it.
   B: I know what you mean. I don't like <u>nosy</u> people.

6. A: News travels fast in this town.
   B: <u>Word of mouth</u> can be very fast.

7. A: I want to give you a <u>heads up</u>.
   B: What's up?
   A: There are going to be some big changes.

8. A: Mrs. Martin sure likes to talk.
   B: I know; I call her <u>motor mouth</u> Martin.

9. A: What do you think of the situation at City Hall?
   B: I don't like it. I <u>smell a rat.</u>

4. Eyes, Ears, and Throat

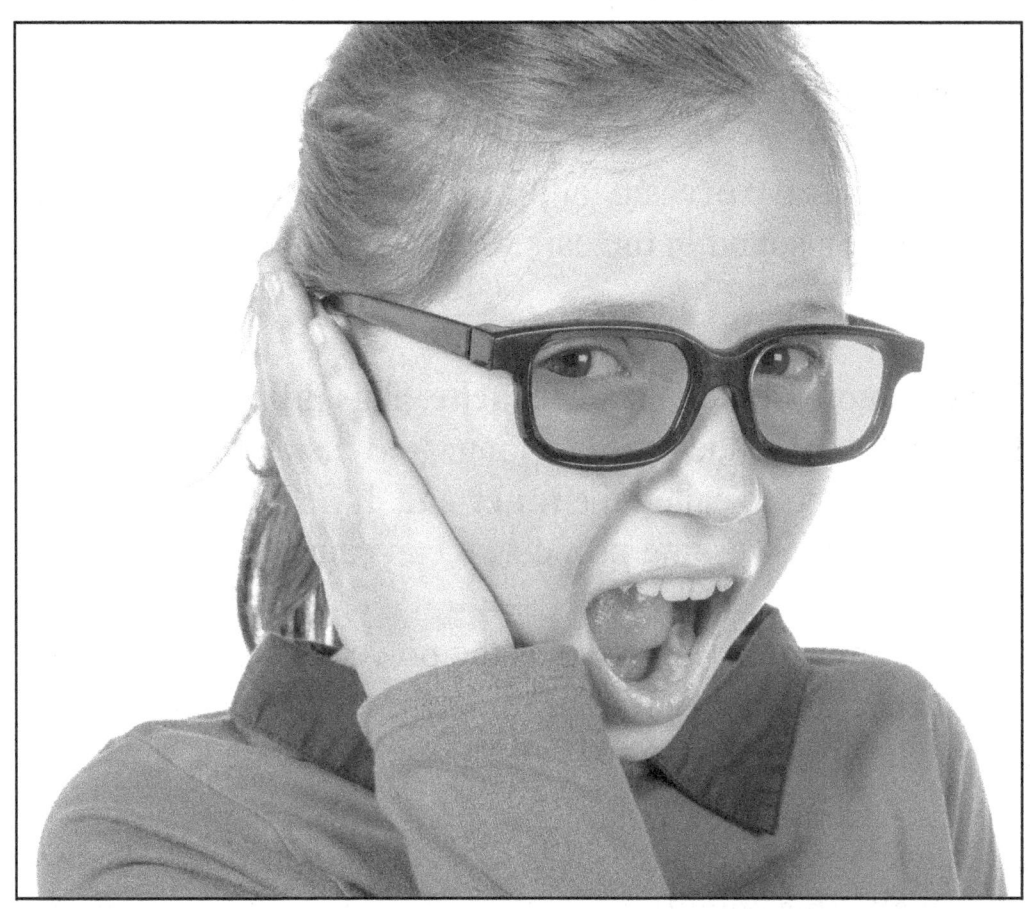

The Earache: Renaud Philippe

Key Words

deaf	blind	mute	ringing ears
tinnitus	earache	inner ear	balance
dizziness	vision	blurry	sore throat
tonsils	infected		

READ

When we have a problem with our eyes or ears, we realize how important they are. Some people are born **deaf** or **blind**. Some are deaf and **mute**, meaning they are unable to hear or speak. These are life-long conditions.

People may also have occasional problems. One common problem is **ringing ears**, a sound in the ears. Often it comes and goes. It is called **tinnitus**.

Another common problem is an **earache**. This problem occurs mostly in children. It does not last long. And inside the ear there is a complex structure called the **inner ear**. It helps us keep our **balance**. If it is not working properly it can cause **dizziness**.

Our eyes are amazing. They give us the power of sight. However, some people do not have good **vison**. What they see is not clear; it is **blurry**. They may need eyeglasses or contact lenses.

Our throat can also give us problems. A common problem is a **sore throat**. Usually this condition is not serious and will go away in a few days. Sometimes two areas in the back of the mouth called the **tonsils** become **infected**. This is tonsillitis. When we have problems with our ear, nose, or throat we should see an ENT specialist. For vision problems, see an eye care professional. *(217)*

EXERCISES
(answers on page 62)

A. Match the two parts of the sentence.

1. People who are deaf _____
2. Ringing ears _____
3. Dizziness can be a problem _____
4. Tonsils can become _____
5. People with poor vision _____
6. He lost his balance _____
7. Children often have _____
8. I don't see well. _____
9. I can't see anything. _____
10. Some people can't speak. _____
11. A sore throat _____

A. and fell down.
B. I am blind.
C. infected.
D. could be tonsillitis.
E. can't hear.
F. with the inner ear.
G. may need glasses.
H. They are mute.
I. is also called tinnitus.
J. Everything is blurry.
K. an earache.

B. Fill in the blanks.

1. If you are _____, you may lose your balance.
2. The _____ is very complex.
3. His _____ is so poor, he is almost blind.
4. My ears are _____ .
5. Ringing ears is another word for _____,
6. The letters on signs are _____;   I don't see them well.
7. Sometimes a deaf person cannot speak; they are _____.
8. My throat is _____.
9. Tonsillitis is an _____ of the _____.
10. Another word for eyesight is _____ .

THINK ABOUT IT
(What is the meaning of the underlined words?)

1. A: So, now do you know why I'm not going?
   B: Yes, I <u>see.</u>

2. A: I've had <u>my eye on</u> that house for months.
   B: And now, it's for sale. Are you going to buy it?

3. A: Alfred! I haven't seen you for months. You're <u>a sight for sore eyes.</u>
   B: And Betty, it's so great to see you, too.

4. A: I can never remember the difference between <u>far-sighted</u> and <u>near-sighted</u>.
   B: If you can see things clearly that are far away, you're <u>far-sighted.</u>

5. A: Look, Mister Jones. I just don't agree with you.
   B: Well, I'm afraid we'll never <u>see eye to eye.</u>

6. A: When Ajaxco announced they were pulling out of the deal, I was <u>blind-sided.</u>
   B: And I had no idea they were thinking about that; I was <u>struck dumb.</u>

7. A: You should join the community chorus.
   B: I can't really sing; I'm <u>tone-deaf.</u>

8. A: Tom's friend is <u>deaf and dumb.</u>
   B: Bill, it's better to say his friend is a <u>deaf-mute.</u>

9. A: A song I heard yesterday is playing over and over in my head.
   B: You've got an <u>earworm.</u> But don't worry; it's not really a worm.

5. The Digestive Tract

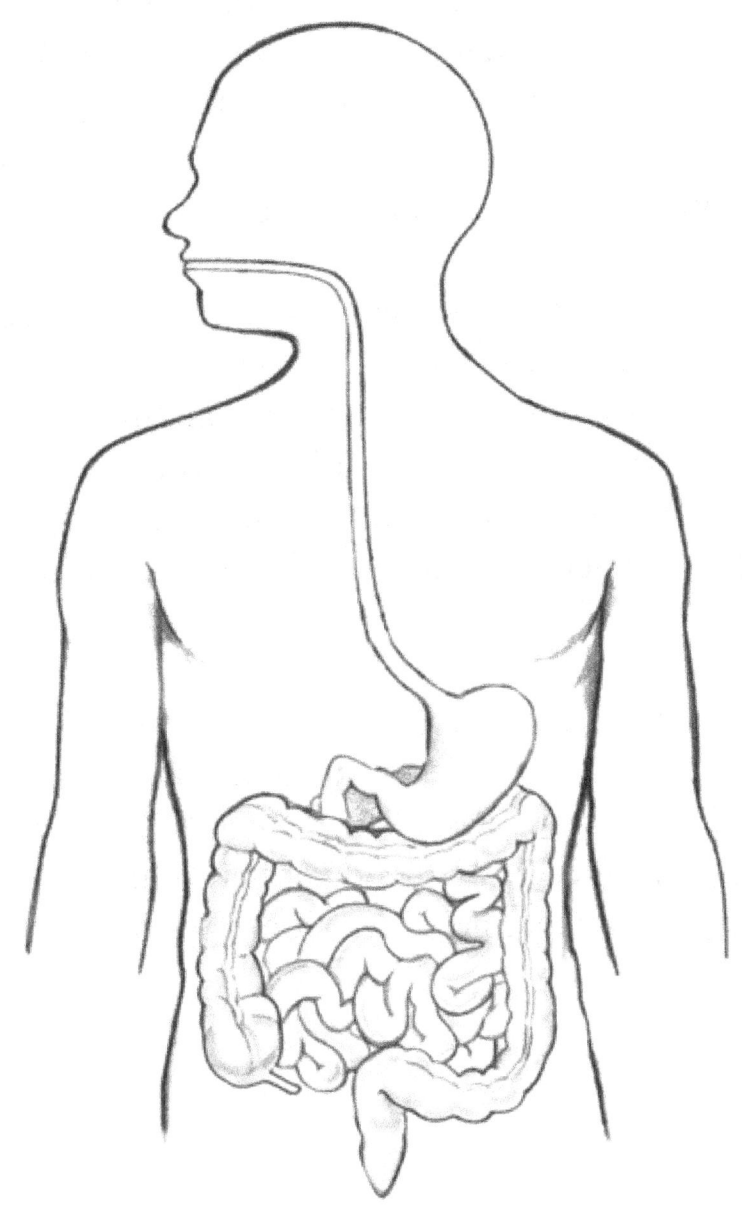

Key Words

to chew	to swallow	throat	esophagus
indigestion	intestine	colon	appendix
anus	diarrhea	rectum	constipation

When we eat something, the food enters the body and goes through the digestive tract. The teeth **chew** the food to make it easy to **swallow,** and in the mouth the digestion of the food begins. The food goes down the **throat** into the **esophagus** and into the stomach. The stomach continues the digestion process, making the food into a kind of soup. Sometimes the process is not comfortable; this is called **indigestion**.

Next the soupy food enters the small **intestine** which continues the digestion. Then the food goes into the large intestine, also called the **colon**. Here water is removed from the food. There is a small organ attached to the colon. It is the **appendix**. It does not seem to have a function, but sometimes the appendix becomes infected. This is called appendicitis. If it bursts, it is a serious problem. It may have to be removed.

Finally, the food leaves the body through the **anus**. Sometimes as the food leaves, it may leave very suddenly, and it is very loose and messy. This is called **diarrhea**. Sometimes it does not leave easily. It stays in the **rectum**, the lower part of the colon. This is called **constipation**. Complete digestion takes one to three days. *(207)*

EXERCISES
(answers on page 62)

A. Match the two parts of the sentence.

1. The food is chewed_____   A. also called the colon.

2. When we swallow_____   B. is the lower part of the colon.

3. The esophagus _____   C. and goes into the small intestine.

4. Indigestion is also called _____ D. the food goes into the throat.

5. The food leaves the stomach _____ E. a common problem.

6. The large intestine is _____   F. in the mouth.

7. An infected appendix_____   G. is like a tube.

8. The rectum _____   H. upset stomach.

9. Diarrhea is_____   I. is dangerous.

B. Fill in the blanks.

1. First, the food is _____ed. Then it is _____ed.

2. The _____ goes into the stomach.

3. _____ means having trouble digesting.

4. The body has two _____s.

5. _____ is a serious problem.

6. The end of the digestive tract is the _____ .

7. What is worse, to have _____ or to be _____?

8. The _____ is the last section of the _____ .

THINK ABOUT IT
(What is the meaning of the underlined words?)

1. A: <u>What's eating you</u>?
   B: Oh, I'm just very worried about the exam.

2. A: Do you need to <u>use the bathroom?</u>
   B: No, I went just a few minutes ago.

3. A: I <u>have a gut feeling</u> something will go wrong.
   B: Relax. Everything is going to be okay.

4. A: Uh oh, the baby's had another <u>BM</u>.
   B: Yeah, I can smell it.

5. A: Boy, am I <u>pissed off.</u>
   B: How come?
   A: My roommate used my toothbrush again.

6. A: My boss really <u>chewed me out.</u>
   B: Why?
   A: I lost my sales report.

7. A: Those two old guys have <u>chewed the fat</u> for at least an hour.
   B: And probably said nothing important.

8. A: Did she believe you?
   B: Yeah, she <u>swallowed it hook, line, and sinker</u>.

9. A: Sorry, but I need <u>to pee.</u>
   B: No problem. There's a gas station up ahead. Anyway, my <u>tummy</u> says it's time for lunch.

6. The Heart, Lungs, and Other Organs

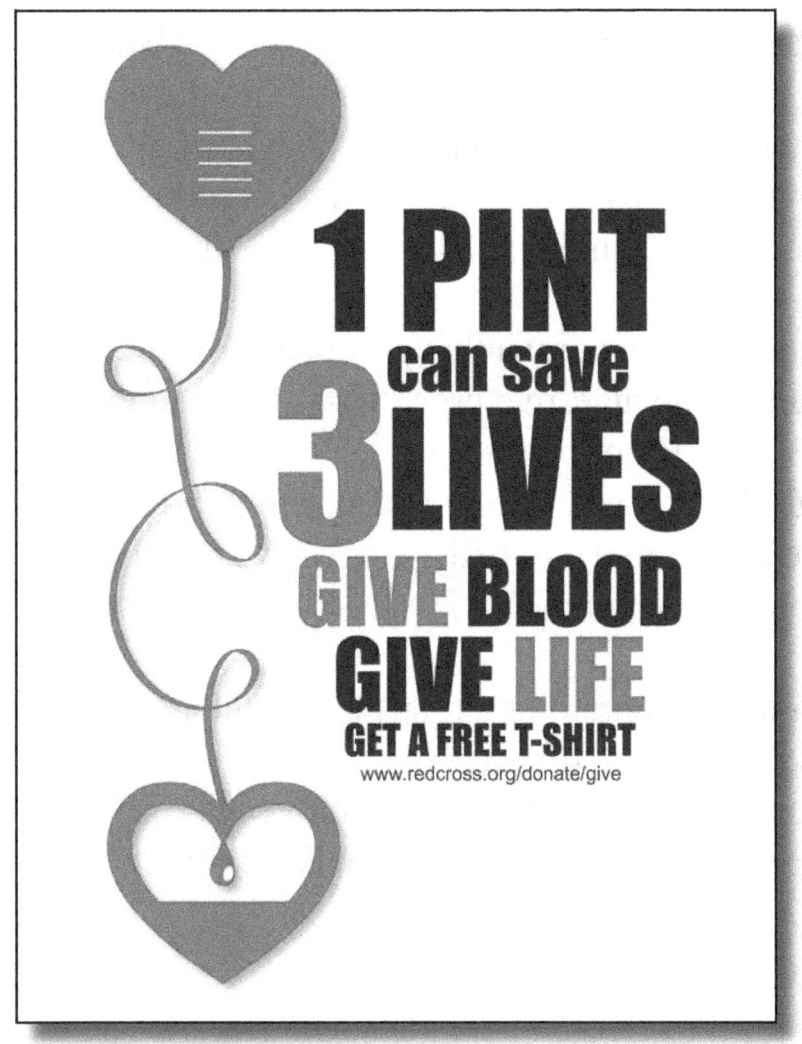

Key Words

to breathe	to inhale	to pump	arteries
to absorb	cells	veins	to exhale
pancreas	enzymes	diabetes	liver
filter	urine	bladder	

The heart and lungs work together along with the digestive system to keep us alive and well. We **breathe** with our lungs. When we breathe, we **inhale** air that has oxygen. This mixture goes into our lungs.

The heart **pumps** blood into our lungs through an **artery**. In the lungs, oxygen becomes **absorbed** into the blood. Then the heart pumps the blood through the body, bringing oxygen to the body's **cells**. **Veins** return the blood with carbon dioxide to the heart and lungs. Finally, the lungs **exhale** the carbon dioxide.

The **pancreas** is an organ that produces **enzymes**, which are important in the digestive process. It also produces **insulin** that controls the level of blood sugar. People who have the disease called **diabetes**, need insulin because their bodies cannot produce and store it. Diabetics must have injections of insulin or use an insulin pump.

There are other important organs inside the body cavity. The **liver** is like a **filter**. It cleans the blood. We also have two kidneys that filter the blood and remove waste. The waste is **urine**, also called pee. It collects in the **bladder** and finally it is urinated. *(192)*

EXERCISES
(answers on page 62)

A. Match the two parts of the sentence.

1. Breathing is _____   A. in the lungs.

2. The liver _____   B. their blood sugar level.

3. Enzymes are produced _____   C. inhaling and exhaling.

4. The heart pumps blood _____   D. by the pancreas.

5. Oxygen is absorbed _____   E. filters the blood.

6. Arteries bring blood _____   F. to the cells.

7. The kidneys remove _____   G. in the bladder.

8. The urine is collected_____   H. urine waste from the blood.

9. Diabetics must watch_____   I. to the lungs.

B. Fill in the blanks.

1. After running hard, he was out of _____.

2. The _____ and _____ filter the blood.

3. _____ carry blood to the heart, and _____ carry it to the _____.

4. When you _____, you bring _____ into the _____.

5. When you _____, you take carbon dioxide out.

6. In the lungs, the blood _____ the oxygen.

7. The pancreas produces _____.

8. The _____ holds _____.

9. There are trillions of _____ in the human body.

10. The heart is like a _____.

CONVERSATION

(With a partner, take turns reading the script from X to Y. Self-studiers, use the audio.)

X Hey, Where ya goin?   To the Veterans Club.

Really? Why?   I'm gonna donate blood.

Why ya doin that?   The Red Cross is havin a blood drive.

What's that?   They're collectin blood for the blood bank.

Blood bank?   The blood is stored at the university medical center.

Why?   There's a daily need for blood. Accidents happen all the time.

Yeah, I guess so.

Can I give blood?   I think so. By the way, what's your blood type?

What dya mean?   Here. Read this. Y

We do not all have the same type of blood. There are four major types: A, B, AB, and O, and each of these types has either a positive or negative Rh-factor. The important point is that if we need blood, most of us cannot receive just any type of blood. There has to be a match, but it is safe to **donate** type O blood to almost anyone. And a person with AB blood type is a universal **recipient**. However, If you have Rh-negative blood, you can only receive Rh-negative blood in a **transfusion**.

---

donate: to give   **recipient**: receiver   **transfusion**: giving and receiving blood

7. Illness, Allergy, and Disease

MOST COMMON INFECTIOUS DISEASES

Chicken pox	Poliomyelitis (polio)
Common cold	Rocky mountain spotted fever
Diphtheria	Rubella (German measles)
E. coli	Salmonella infections
Giardiasis	Severe acute respiratory
HIV/AIDS	syndrome (SARS)
Infectious mononucleosis	Sexually transmitted diseases
Influenza (flu)	Shingles (herpes zoster)
Lyme disease	Tetanus
Malaria	Toxic shock syndrome
Measles	Tuberculosis
Meningitis	Viral hepatitis
Mumps	West Nile virus
Pneumonia	Whooping cough (pertussis)

Source: https://healthcare.utah.edu/infectiousdiseases/general.php

Key Words

sprain	to twist	ankle	fracture
rash	to cough	to sneeze	runny
heart attack	pneumonia	tuberculosis	symptoms
epidemic	pandemic	cancer	

READ

Being and staying healthy is not always easy or possible. Many things can go wrong with our body, resulting in discomfort or an illness. Some problems are accidental or the result of carelessness–for example, a sunburn, staying too long unprotected from sunshine. Sometimes a painful **sprain** is the result of **twisting** an **ankle**. When we twist or bend a leg or arm too far and the bone breaks, that is a **fracture**.

Another common problem for many people is an allergy. Some people get a **rash** on their skin because they are allergic to a poisonous plant. For some people, breathing air that has allergens causes **coughing** and **sneezing**, and **runny** eyes and nose.

A disease, however, can be more serious and cause death. Heart disease can result in a sudden life-threatening **heart attack**. **Pneumonia** and **tuberculosis** are diseases of the lungs. The flu, with **symptoms** of the common cold, can be dangerous. It attacks the lungs, nose, and throat. It can become an **epidemic**, meaning it is very widespread. An epidemic can become a **pandemic**, affecting the entire world. The COVID-19 pandemic has killed many people in every country.

Possibly the most feared disease that affects both children and adults is **cancer**. After heart disease, it is the leading cause of death in the United States. *(220)*

EXERCISES
(answers on page 63)

A. Match the two parts of the sentence.

1. Twisting an ankle_____   A. may become a pandemic.
2. She fractured_____   B. can be serious.
3. Coughing _____   C. attacks the lungs.
4. Allergens can cause _____   D. coughing and sneezing.
5. If you have a runny nose, _____ E. you may have an allergy.
6. Heart attacks _____   F. a leg bone.
7. Pneumonia_____   G. can be itchy.
8. An epidemic_____   H. often results in a sprain.
9. A skin rash_____   I. can be a symptom of the flu.

B. Fill in the blanks.

1. _____ is also called TB.
2. The worst disease is _____.
3. Another word for "break" is _____.
4. COVID-19 is a _____.
5. She _____ ed her _____ while she was running.
6. Poison ivy caused my itchy _____.
7. When you _____ or _____, cover your nose and mouth.
8. Her son had the _____, not a common cold.
9. It wasn't easy to breathe; it was _____.
10. Chest pains are a _____ of heart disease.

THINK ABOUT IT
(What is the meaning of the underlined words?)

1. A: I was <u>sick as a dog</u> last week.
   B: What happened?
   A: I don't know, but I was <u>bed-ridden</u> for four days, and I <u>ran a fever</u> of 102°.

2. A: Let's go for a walk.
   B: Can't.
   A: Why not?
   B: I've got <u>the runs</u>, and I've gotta stay close to the toilet.

3. A: You look angry.
   B: I am. I'm <u>sick and tired</u> of listening to political nonsense.

4. A: I've gotta go home.
   B: How come?
   A: I'm just feeling <u>lousy.</u>
   B: I hope you're not <u>coming down with</u> the flu. Let me <u>take your temperature</u>.

5. A: Spring is here!
   B: And I'<u>m itching to</u> play golf again.

6. A: The senator looks very <u>ill at ease</u>.
   B: He should be; he's lying.

7. A: Why isn't their ace pitcher playing?
   B: He's <u>nursing</u> a sore arm.

8. A: It sounds like you've got the <u>sniffles</u>.
   B: Yeah, I know. I'm sneezing and my <u>nose is running</u>.

8. The Doctor's Office

Middle Village Family Medicine
215 Main Street
Middle Village, OH

NAME _____   DOB _____
       Last   First   MI   Insurance _____

HOME ADDRESS   WORK ADDRESS
Street _____   Company _____
City _____   Street _____
State _____ ZIP _____   City _____
                                       State _____ ZIP _____

Telephone _____   Telephone _____
Cell Phone _____

Emergency Contact Name _____
Telephone _____
Address _____ City _____ State ____ ZIP ____

Known allergies

Current medications   Blood type

Surgeries   Reason for visit

Key Words

healthcare provider	primary care	specialist	clinic
receptionist	appointment	waiting room	urgent
emergency	examination room	weight	height
blood pressure	to prescribe		

READ

Sometimes we need to see a person who can help us with a medical problem. Most people have a **healthcare provider** who gives **primary care**. This person is often a doctor, but they may be a Physican Assistant or Nurse Practitioner. These professionals help you directly and may refer you to a **specialist** for additional help.

These healthcare professionals may work in a private office or in a **clinic** or in a hospital. In a clinic there may be more than one "doctor" as well as nurses, medical assistants, and a **receptionist**.

To visit a doctor, you usually need to make an **appointment**. When you go for your appointment, a receptionist is the first person you see. They will ask for your basic information, ask about your insurance, and ask you to have a seat in the **waiting room**. Sometimes the problem is **urgent**, an **emergency**, and you need help immediately. In this case, go directly to the ER, the emergency room, at a hospital.

When it is your turn to see the healthcare provider, a nurse or medical assistant will take you to an **examination room**. They will check your **weight**, **height**, and **blood pressure**. Then the healthcare provider will see you. If they think a medicine would be helpful, they will **prescribe** a medicine. They write a prescription and send it to your pharmacy. *(226)*

EXERCISES
(answers on page 63)

A. Match the two parts of the sentence.

1. A healthcare provider_____   A. will greet you at the office.

2. Primary care _____   B. healthcare providers in a clinic.

3. A specialist _____   C. a prescription.

4. A receptionist _____   D. you do not make an appointment.

5. First, you should _____   E. take your blood pressure.

6. A nurse may_____   F. make an appointment.

7. If there is an emergency,____   G. is basic health care.

8. There may be several _____   H. helps patients.

9. They will write _____   I. works with specific health

                                        problems.

B. Fill in the blanks.

1. A _____ provider gives primary care.

2. First you wait in the _____.

   Then you go to the _____.

3. You make an _____ with a _____.

4. An assistant will take your blood _____ .

5. You are _____ weight. You need to eat less.

6. If you need _____ care, go to the

   _____ room.

7. She will _____ a stronger medicine.

8. I can't help you with this. You need to see a _____.

CONVERSATION

(Practice the conversation with a partner. A begins.)

A	**B**
Good morning, may I help you? And your name is?	I have an appointment to see Dr. Cho. _____.

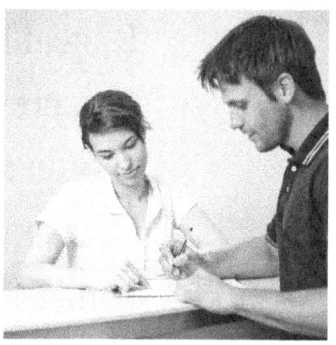

_____, please fill this out and have a seat in the waiting room. Dr. Cho's assistant will see you soon.	Thank you.

****

_____?	Yes. Here.
Hello, _____, please come with me.	Okay.
Here we are at the examination room. Please sit here. Let's take your blood pressure. , , , , ,	How is it?
It's 120 over 80.	Is that good?
Yes, that's normal. Now step up here. We'll take your weight.	It's 180, I think.
Yes, 182. And your height is 5-6.	I have shoes on.
Yes, I know. But your BMI is 29. That's a little overweight.	Oh, I know.
You can discuss that with Dr.Cho. She'll be with you in a moment.	

9. At the Dentist

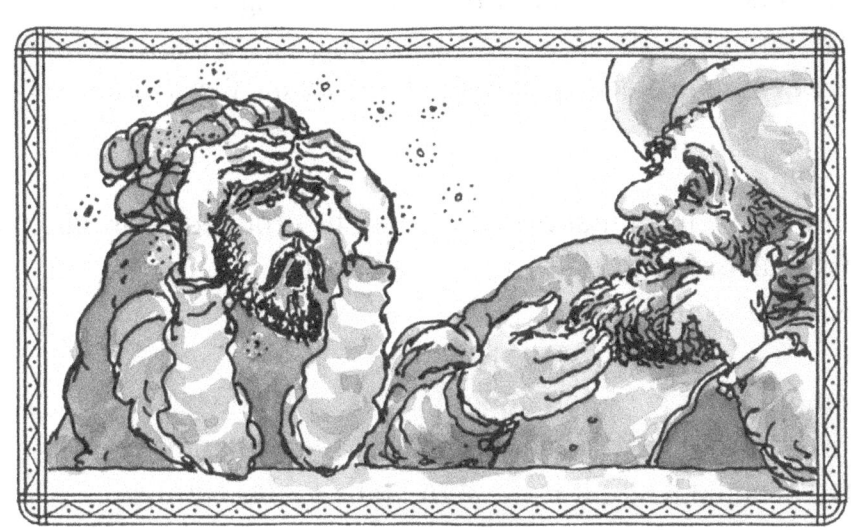

There was a man who often asked Hodja for advice. Usually Hodja thought the man's problems were not very important. One day he came to Hodja with this problem: "I have a headache. What should I do?"

Hodja replied, "I'm not sure, my friend, but I can tell you that recently I had a toothache. I had the tooth pulled out, and it doesn't bother me now."

Nasreddin Hodja: Raymond C. Clark/ Robert MacLean

Key Words

gum	permanent	orthodontist	braces
to brush	to floss	hygienist	to decay
cavity	to drill	filling	to inject
medication	syringe	needle	root canal
crown	to extract		

READ

When we are born, our teeth are inside our **gums**. We look like we have no teeth. When we are about 6 months old, these teeth begin to grow out of our gums. This can be painful. It is called "cutting one's teeth." By 30 to 36 months we will have 20 "baby teeth." At age 6, we begin to lose our baby teeth and **permanent** teeth will begin to grow in. We will have 32 permanent teeth.

As our teeth grow in, sometimes they may be crooked. Our parents may consult with an **orthodontist**. They may decide to have the child wear **braces** on their teeth.

Taking care of teeth is important and necessary. The basic care is **brushing** the teeth with a toothbrush and toothpaste. **Floss** may be used to clean the spaces between the teeth. It is good to do this after eating.

It is normal for people to see their dentist every six months. At the dentist's office, the dental **hygienist** will check and clean the teeth. They will sometimes take an x-ray to see if the teeth are healthy. Sometimes a tooth can become unhealthy. An infected tooth, a toothache, can be painful. There will be a place that is **decaying**. This is called a **cavity**. The dentist will use a **drill** to remove the bad part of the tooth. After that, the dentist will put a **filling** in the tooth. Dental work can be painful. A local anesthetic (lidocaine) is used. The dentist **injects** the **medication** using a **syringe** and **needle**.

A tooth can become very infected, and then the dentist has to remove the inside part of the tooth. This is called a **root canal**. After the decayed material has been removed, the tooth may need a **crown**. This is like a cap on top of the tooth to protect and strengthen it. Sometimes a tooth cannot be saved. Then it is necessary to **extract** the tooth. *(324)*

EXERCISES
(answers on page 63)

A. Match the two parts of the sentence.

1. Our baby teeth _____	A. it begins to decay.
2. We wear braces _____	B. to clean between teeth.
3. We should brush our teeth _____	C. may need a root canal.
4. When a tooth is infected, _____	D. an anesthetic is used.
5. Use floss _____	E. be injected.
6. A cavity _____	F. are inside our gums at birth.
7. The dentist will _____	G. to straighten our teeth.
8. To reduce pain, _____	H. is like a hole.
9. A badly infected tooth _____	I. fill the cavity.
10. A crown _____	J. after eating.
11. Medication will _____	K. protects the tooth.

B. Fill in the blanks.

1. Dental work may require an _____.

2. Teeth are cleaned with a _____ and _____.

3. _____ can straighten crooked teeth.

4. _____ is injected.

5. Teeth grow in the _____.

6. A _____ may take an x-ray.

7. _____ is reduced with a needle and _____.

8. An _____ tooth has been _____ from the gum.

9. A _____ may need a crown.

10. The dentist said the tooth was badly _____.

THINK ABOUT IT
(What is the meaning of the underlined words?)

1. A: How did you win the game? They were a strong team.
   B: We just fought <u>tooth and nail</u>.

2. A: Look at that SuperSedan 1500. What a beautiful car!
   B: I'd <u>give my eyeteeth</u> for one of those.

3. A: I'm afraid that molar needs to be extracted.
   B: You mean <u>pull it out</u>? Oh, no!

4. A: You should place your baby tooth under your pillow tonight.
   B: Why? What will happen?
   A: The <u>tooth fairy</u> will leave some money for it.

5. A: You ate that whole bag of cookies.
   B: I know, I have a real <u>sweet tooth</u>.

6. A: This proposal is worth over a million dollars.
   B: Be careful. Taking on that project could be <u>biting off more than we can chew.</u>

7. A: Did you hear what she just said? That is not true.
   B: I did. What could I do? I just had to <u>bite my tongue</u>.

8. A: Every night I have to push Dickie to do his homework.
   B: Know what you mean. Same with Stevie. It's <u>like pulling teeth</u>.

9. A: I can't wait to <u>sink my teeth into</u> this project.
   B: Me, too. I'm ready to go right now.

10. A: Millie has such a nice smile.
    B: But did you know she has <u>false teeth</u>?
    A: Yes, I did. So what?

10. The Hospital

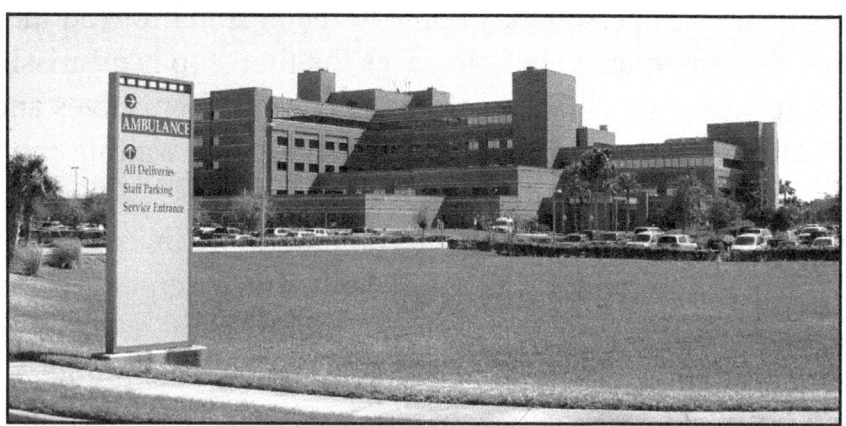

MIDDLETOWN GENERAL HOSPITAL
DIRECTORY

Anesthesiology D7	Outpatient Surgery A4
Audiology B6	Parkinson's Disease Center A5
Cardiovascular Medicine D2	Pediatric Cancer B5
Dermatology C9	Pharmacy A2
Emergency A3	Plastic Surgery D3
Cancer Center C1	Podiatry B2
Infectious Disease B5	Psychiatry D8
Internal Medicine C6	Pulmonary Medicine C3
Laboratory Services B3	Radiology B3
Multiple Sclerosis Center C9	Rheumatology B1
Hernia Surgery Center D4	Sports Concussion Program A7
Neurology C5	Surgery Department D1
OB/GYN B8	Surgical Oncology D2
Ophthalmology C2	Trauma Program A2
Orthopaedics B7	Urology C8

Key Words

admissions	ambulance	severe	radiology
x-ray	CT scan	tumor	MRI
lab(oratory)	maternity	delivery room	operating room
to anesthetize	surgery	ICU	outpatient

READ

The hospital is a large and busy place. It provides many services to help people stay healthy. A person may come to the hospital for routine care or because of an emergency. In both cases the first stop is **admissions**. At admissions, patients will give information about themselves and their insurance. The admissions people then send them to a waiting room.

Sometimes people have a very urgent problem. Sometimes a person has had an accident. They cannot wait to get help. The emergency room takes people when they have an urgent problem. Some people walk in. Some come in an **ambulance** or rescue vehicle. Sometimes the problem is **severe**, and a small hospital sends the patient to a larger hospital by helicopter.

There are many other places that provide help. If a problem is about a bone, the patient will go to the **radiology** department for an **x-ray**. Other internal problems may require examination by a large machine. This examination is called a **CT scan** or CAT scan. It can see fractures, **tumors**, and fluid collections like blood. Another kind of machine does an **MRI** exam. It can sometimes see things a CT scan cannot.

Sometimes a doctor may want their patient to have a blood test. The person goes to a place in the hospital for a blood test. This place is called the **laboratory**, often called "the lab," and the tests are called "labs."

Hospitals also have a section called **maternity**. This is where women give birth to babies. This is done in the **delivery** room. Hospitals allow the father to be in the delivery room.

One part of the hospital is the **operating room** (OR). The surgeon needs to open a place in the body where there is a problem. The patient is **anesthetized** by an anesthesiologist. They do not feel any pain. After the **surgery**, the patent may stay in the hospital. Severe cases may go to an intensive Care Unit (**ICU**). Patients with mInor surgery can be **outpatients** and leave the hospital after the surgery. *(342)*

EXERCISES

(answers on page 64)

A. Match the two parts of the sentence.

1. The first stop_____	A. works in the OR.
2. She came to the hospital _____	B. does not stay in the hospital.
3. You can get an x-ray _____	C. severe?
4. A CT scan _____	D. does not feel pain.
5. An MRI can see _____	E. in an ambulance.
6. My doctor ordered_____	F. in the maternity section.
7. Babies are delivered_____	G. at the radiology department.
8. A surgeon _____	H. can detect a fractured bone or tumor.
9. An anesthetized patient _____	I. labs.
10. An outpatient _____	J. more than a CT scan.
11. Is your pain _____	K. is admissions.

B. Fill in the blanks.

1. The _____ is in the maternity section.

2. Surgery is done in the _____ room.

3. An _____ does not stay overnight.

4. Someone in _____ will tell you where to go.

5. X-rays are done at the _____ department.

6. An _____ is given by an anesthesiologist.

7. Surgery is performed by a _____.

8. The doctor asked if my pain was _____.

9. The MRI showed a _____ in the abdomen.

10. The _____ raced through the streets.

11. The CT _____ did not show anything.

12. The surgery was successful, and your friend is now in the _____ unit.

CONVERSATION

(Practice the conversation with a partner.)

DOCTOR	PATIENT
Good morning. I'm Doctor _____, and you must be _____.	That's right.
So your hand is giving you a problem? Which hand?	
	Left.
Let's take a look. Hmmm, I can see some swelling around the middle knuckle. How long has it been like this?	
	About six weeks.
Are you feeling any pain?	At first I didn't notice, but now it hurts when I make a fist.
On a scale of one to ten, ten being severe, how do you rate it?	I'd say six or seven.
What have you been taking for the pain?	Ibuprofen.
Has it helped?	Some.
OK. We'll need to take some x-rays. I'll set you up for radiology.	Do I go there now?
Yes. It's on level 2. I'll be in touch later after I've seen the x-rays.	Soon, I hope.
Probably tomorrow.	OK. Thank you.
Nice meeting you.	Nice to meet you, too, Doctor _____.

11. Nutrition

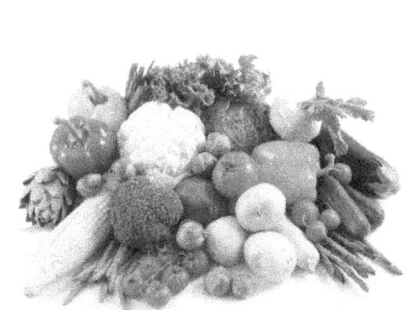

12 Best Vegetables

1. spinach
2. carrot
3. broccoli
4. garlic
5. Brussels sprouts
6. kale
7. green peas
8. Swiss chard
9. ginger
10. asparagus
11. red cabbage
12. sweet potato

Source: healthline.com

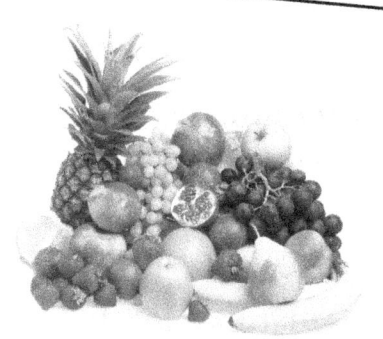

12 Best Fruits

1. lemon
2. strawberry
3. orange
4. lime
5. grapefruit
6. blackberry
7. apple
8. pomegranate
9. pineapple
10. banana
11. avocado
12. blueberry

Source: medicalnewstoday.com

Key Words

balanced diet	grains	protein	nutritionist
calorie	nutrient	carbohydrate	vitamin
mineral	muscles	starch	fiber
processed	quantity	obese	

Staying healthy means eating healthy, and that means eating a **balanced diet** of food and drinks. A balanced diet includes **grains**, vegetables, fruit, dairy, and foods that include **protein**.

Nutritionists can tell us which foods are the most nutritious or the best ones for us.   We also need to know which foods can give us energy. Food is like fuel for us, just as a machine needs fuel. Our "fuel" gives us energy, and it is measured in **calories.** Too many or too few calories are not good. The average man needs 2,500 calories every day; the average woman needs 2,000.

Nutritious food provides **nutrients** for our body. These nutrients include protein, **carbohydrates**, fat, water, **vitamins**, and **minerals**. Protein builds **muscles**. We get protein from meat, fish, eggs, and beans. The three main types of carbohydrates are sugar, **starches**, and **fiber**. Carbohydrates can be healthy or unhealthy. Healthy carbohydrates can be found in grains, vegetables, fruits, and beans. They promote good health by delivering vitamins, minerals, and fiber. Unhealthy foods with carbohydrates include **processed** foods such as cereals, chips, cookies, and frozen dinners.

Eating well also means we need to watch the **quantity** of food we eat. Eating too much can make us fat and even **obese**. What and how much we eat is important. *(215)*

EXERCISES
(answers on page 64)

A. Match the two parts of the sentence.

1. A balanced diet includes_____   A. healthy carbohydrates.
2. Protein builds_____   B. processed food.
3. We can get protein _____   C. is very important.
4. Starch_____   D. needs about 2,000 calories.
5. Grains are_____   E. is one kind of carbohydrate.
6. Cereal is a_____   F. our muscles.
7. The quantity of food we eat _____   G. is too fat.
8. An obese person _____   H. are nutrients.
9. Vitamins and minerals_____   I. many kinds of foods.
10. The average woman_____   J. from eggs.

B. Fill in the blanks.

1. A _____ can tell us about a balanced_____.
2. Our food intake is measured in _____.
3. There are three main types of _____.
4. Sugar, _____, and fiber are carbohydrates.
5. Processed foods often are not very _____.
6. Protein helps build _____.
7. An _____ person probably eats too much food.
8. The quality and _____ of food we eat is very important.

CONVERSATION

(Read the script with a partner.)

A	**B**
_____! I haven't seen you for weeks. How are you?	Fit as a fiddle. And how about you?
I've been down in the dumps recently.	What's going on?
Oh, stress at work, for one thing. And to be honest, I'm not eating well. I haven't been watching my diet and I've put on a few pounds.	I noticed. What plan are you following?
Doctor Feelwell's.	Hmm. I've heard of it. Low-carb, Right?
Yes, But really, I'm not sticking to the regimen. Too many snacks at work.	Not good. Why don't you join my H & E group?
H & E?	Health and exercise. We walk Tuesdays and Thursdays, but we talk a lot about our diets.
Do you have a plan?	Yes, but I'm also a vegetarian, so it's a little heavy on protein. You're a meat eater, aren't you?
Yes, but I try to avoid red meat.	Good idea. Why don't you come to Wellness Club this Tuesday?
I'll think about it.	Don't think, do it!

12. Exercise

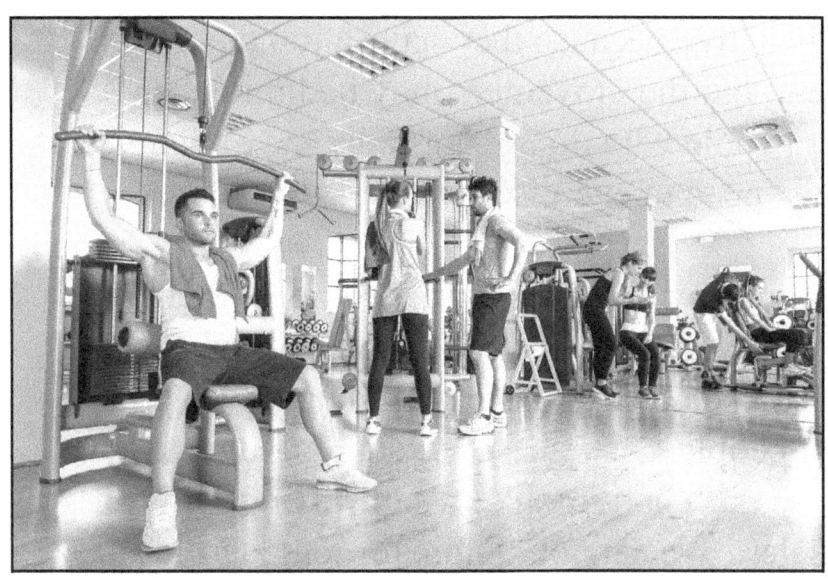

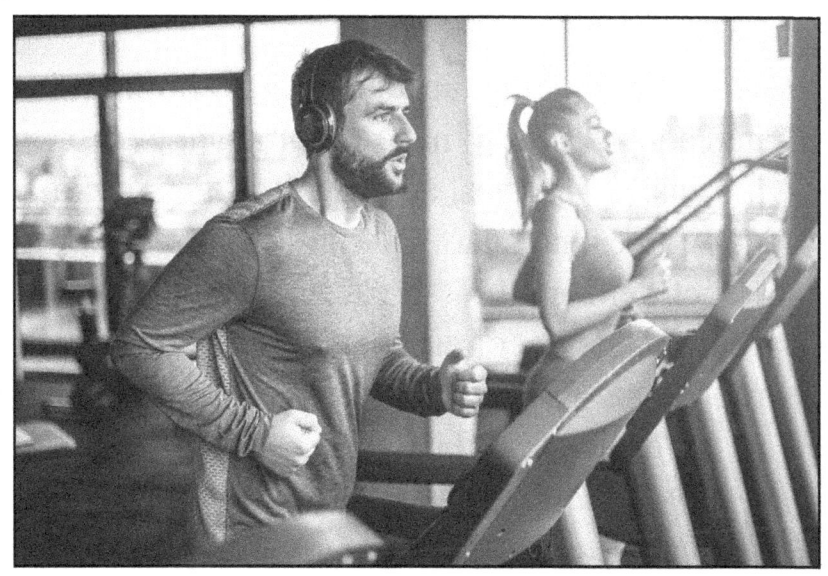

Key Words

aerobic	anaerobic	jogging	weightlifting
intensive	weight loss	cardiovascular	benefits
risk	fitness	gym	routine

READ

Staying healthy means eating well, and it means being active. Our body needs to be used. As the old saying goes, "Use it or lose it." Some people are naturally active because they have a job that requires a lot of movement, but the movement may be limited. For those people, and for people who do not normally move their bodies during the day, they need to exercise.

There are two kinds of exercise: **aerobic** and **anaerobic**. Aerobic exercise includes walking, swimming, **jogging**, running, and cycling. These activities can be done for several minutes, even hours. For example, most people can walk for twenty minutes or longer. Anaerobic exercise is an activity like **weightlifting**. It is an **intensive** use of our muscles. We cannot do this for long periods of time. Both types are useful, but for **weight loss**, aerobic is better.

Walking, jogging, and running do not require special equipment, but it is a good idea to have running shoes. For most people, walking is the easiest and best activity. It is a **cardiovascular** activity, meaning it involves the heart and blood vessels. Aerobic activities have many **benefits** in addition to cardiovascular **fitness**. Walking can improve some kinds of conditions, such as minor arthritis pain. It can also reduce the **risk** of heart disease and stroke and help us maintain stronger bones and balance.

Anaerobic exercise has many benefits. It burns fat, and builds and maintains muscles, which makes us stronger. Many people have exercise equipment at home or join a **fitness** club or **gym** that has many kinds of equipment. A very simple piece of equipment is a set of barbells. They are not only easy to use, they are inexpensive. Whatever kind of exercise you choose to do, the really important thing is to establish a **routine** and keep doing it. *(304)*

EXERCISES
(answers on page 64)

A. Match the two parts of the sentence.

1. There are two kinds _____   A. a cardiovascular activity.
2. Aerobic exercise includes _____   B. can be reduced.
3. Weightlifting is an _____   C. has many kinds of equipment.
4. An anaerobic activity _____   D. minor arthritic pain.
5. For weight loss _____   E. is one of the benefits of exercise.
6. Swimming is _____   F. anaerobic activity.
7. Walking can improve _____   G. is a good length for a routine.
8. The risk of heart disease _____   H. involves intensive use of muscles.
9. A gym _____   I. swimming and walking.
10. Twenty minutes every day _____   J. aerobics is better than anaerobics.
11. Maintaining stronger bones _____ K. of exercise.

B. Fill in the blanks.

1. _____ and _____ are two kinds of exercise.
2. An anaerobic activity can be _____ lifting.
3. Jogging is an _____ activity.
4. Anaerobics strengthen our _____ .
5. The _____ of heart disease can be reduced by exercising.
6. A _____ club is also known as a _____.
7. Aerobic activity is better for losing _____.
8. A daily exercise _____ is very beneficial.

Establish a Weekly Routine

DAY/DATE	ACTIVITY	BEGIN TIME	END TIME	DONE (√)
MON				
TUE				
WED				
THU				
FRI				
SAT				
SUN				

A

Have you done your exercise routine chart?

Why not?

That's a poor excuse.

No "buts." Just fill it out.

So, get ...

Tomorrow's too late.

OK, Let's see. It's Monday. So fill out the chart.

B

No, not yet.

I've been busy.

Yeah, I know, but...

All right already!

Right, right, right. I'll start tomorrow.

All right. Let's go for a walk.

Now? I wanna walk.

13. Mental Health

THE FIVE MOST COMMON TYPES OF MENTAL DISORDER

Anxiety disorders, which include
      obsessive-compulsive syndrome
      panic
      post-traumatic stress
Mood disorders
      depression
      bipolar disorder
      substance-induced mood disorder
Psychotic disorders
      schizophrenia
      delusional disorder
      substance-induced psychotic disorder
Dementia, including
      Alzheimer's disease
      Parkinson's disease
Eating disorders
      anorexia
      bulimia
      binge eating

Source: Davis Behavioral Health. www.dbhutah.org

Key Words

to cope	normal	stress	productively
to suffer	disorder	chronic	substance abuse
psychotic	addiction	preventable	to quit
alcoholism			

When a person is mentally healthy they know their strengths and weaknesses, and they can **cope** with the normal **stresses** of life. They can work **productively** and are able to make a contribution to their community.

When a person is mentally ill, they have problems with reality. This means they can't cope with the normal stresses of life, they lose productivity, and they are not participating successfully in their community.

A mentally ill person is **suffering** from a mental **disorder**. The disorder may be occasional or **chronic**, lasting a lifetime. There may be ways to limit or control a disorder, but some may need professional help.

Related to mental disorders is another very serious health problem: **substance abuse,** which can lead to mood and **psychotic** disorders. Substance abuse often results in **addiction**. One common addiction is to the nicotine in tobacco, caused by smoking cigarettes. Fortunately, tobacco addiction is **preventable**. **Quitting** is not easy, but many people do it .

Perhaps the most common substance abuse is "drinking too much," or **alcoholism**. Many people drink alcohol and do not become alcoholic, meaning their drinking does not interfere with their lives. They do not become addicted, and they can easily go through several days without needing to drink. An alcoholic, however, has a much harder time and may need the help of an organization that helps people with their addictions.

Drug addiction has always been around. Drugs like cocaine and heroin can be very dangerous and addictive. Prescription drugs such as opioids and amphetamines are a new problem, and the use of drugs has also led to an increase in crime. *(271)*

EXERCISES
(answers on page 65)

A. Match the two parts of the sentence.

1. A mentally healthy person_____	A. is preventable.
2. A friend of mine _____	B. the nicotine in tobacco.
3. She is suffering _____	C. for years. It is chronic.
4. She has had the problem _____	D. can work productively.
5. Substance abuse can lead to _____	E. to quit smoking.
6. Many people are addicted to _____	F. drinking too much alcohol.
7. Drug addiction_____	G. has problems with reality.
8. It was difficult _____	H. a psychotic disorder.
9. Alcoholism is _____	I. from a mental disorder.

B. Fill in the blanks.

1. He _____from drug _____.

2. There are many kinds of mental _____s.

3. She cannot _____ with _____.

4. _____ abuse is a dangerous problem.

5. Mentally unhealthy people are usually not _____.

6. He said, "It's very easy to _____. I do it every day."

7. The problem continues; it is _____.

8. A person who is addicted to alcohol is an _____.

9. A severe mental illness is a _____.

10. An ounce of _____ is worth a pound of cure.

THINK ABOUT IT

(Make a list of ten words in this reading that you are not sure about. Compare your list with a friend. Then together find out the meanings.)

ANXIETY*

Anxiety disorders are the most common mental illness in the United States, affecting 40 million adults age 18 and older, or 18.1% of the population every year.

- Anxiety disorders are highly treatable, yet only 36.9% of those suffering receive treatment.
- People with an anxiety disorder are three to five times more likely to go to the doctor and six times more likely to be hospitalized for psychiatric disorders than those who do not suffer from anxiety disorders.
- Anxiety disorders develop from a complex set of risk factors, including genetics, brain chemistry, personality, and life events.

It's not uncommon for someone with an anxiety disorder to also suffer from depression or vice versa. Nearly one-half of those diagnosed with depression are also diagnosed with an anxiety disorder.

* Source: Anxiety and Depression Association of America (ADAA)

---

1. _____

2. _____

3. _____

4. _____

5. _____

6. _____

7. _____

8. _____

9. _____

10. _____

14. Public Health

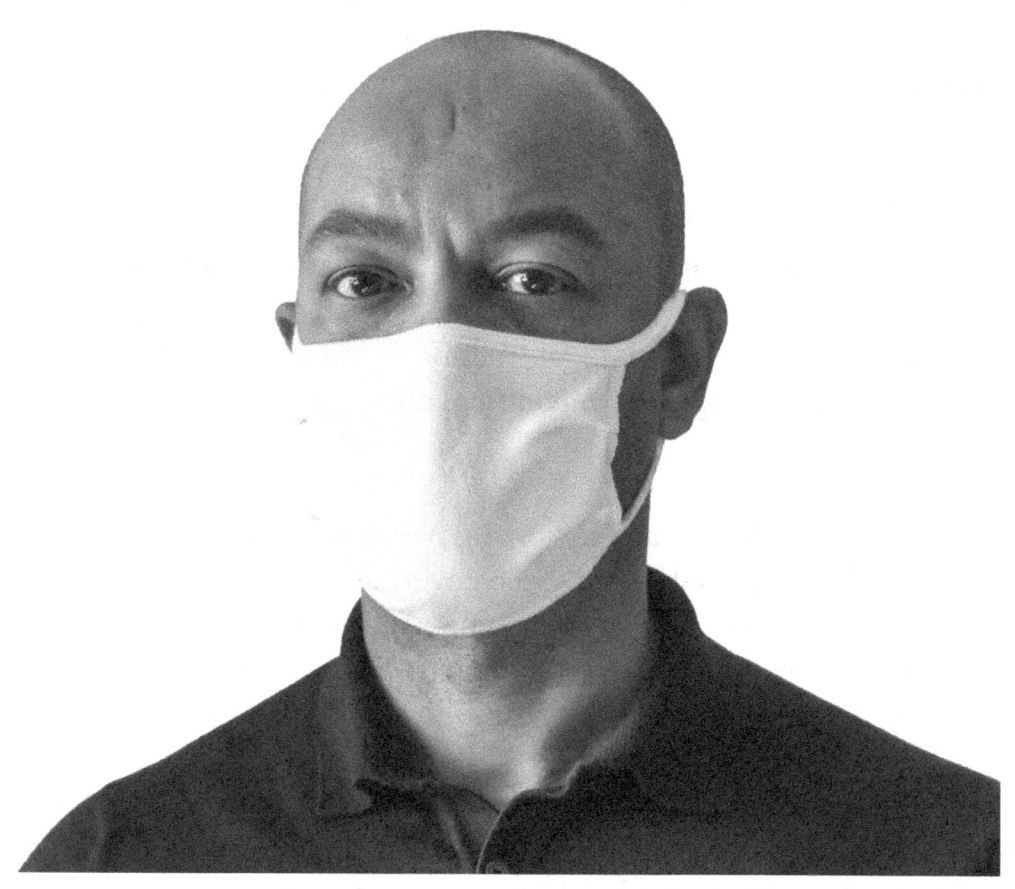

Key Words

to maintain	collective	infectious	contagious
to contain	spread	virus	crisis
pharmaceutical	vaccine	protective	to peak
herd immunity			

READ

Personal health is about individuals **maintaining** good health. Public health, however, is about the **collective** health of a community, of everyone in a place. When an **infectious** and very **contagious** disease affects many people and becomes an epidemic, the disease **spreads**, and it can affect a nation, or even many nations. When this happens, it is called a pandemic, and public health agencies try to **contain** the spread of the disease.

In 2019 a new infectious **virus** began to spread from a city in China. It spread to a much larger community and then on to entire nations. It became an international **crisis**. In the United States, the CDC (Centers for Disease Control and Prevention) began to take action. It identified the nature of the disease and asked leading **pharmaceutical** companies to begin researching for a **vaccine**.

The CDC, acting with state and national governments, began recommending that public policies be established. Face coverings such as masks were required in public places. Social distancing was put in place. Large quantities of personal **protective** equipment were ordered and distributed. Educational campaigns urged people to follow the guidelines and policies.

The national death toll in the United States **peaked** in January of 2021. Then, as more and more people became vaccinated, the spread of the disease slowed down. In some places **herd immunity** was established simply because the disease had fewer and fewer targets. However, COVID-19 still exists. *(236)*

EXERCISES
(answers on page 65)

A. Match the two parts of the sentence.

1. The CDC's mission _____	A. can be caused by a virus.
2. The epidemic became _____	B. personal protective equipment.
3. Collective health _____	C. can be passed from person to person.
4. An infectious disease _____	D. establish herd immunity.
5.The crisis _____	E. been vaccinated.
6. Hospitals needed more_____	F. is to maintain good community health.
7. A contagious disease_____	G. the spread of the disease.
8. A pharmaceutical company _____	H. refers to the health of a community.
9. 50% of the state has_____	I. peaked in January.
10. Vaccinations helped contain _____	J. a pandemic.
11. Social distancing helped _____	K. created vaccines.

B. Fill in the blanks.

1. _____ prevented the disease from spreading.

2. A _____ disease spreads very rapidly.

3. COVID-19 is an _____ disease.

4. _____ good health is very important for everyone.

5.Tbe Centers for Disease Control and _____ is in Atlanta.

6. The health _____ reached a peak in the winter.

7. If you are vaccinated, you are _____.

8. Masks are a simple form of _____ equipment.

9. A very dangerous _____ caused the disease.

RESEARCH

(Find out what all these names, titles, and acronyms are.)

COVID   _____

CDC   _____

WHO   _____

FDA   _____

HHS   _____

MD   _____

RN   _____

LPN   _____

PA   _____

NP   _____

DO   _____

ENT   _____

BMI   _____

BP   _____

CPR   _____

DNR   _____

EKG   _____

MRI   _____

OR   _____

PT   _____

15. Birth and Death

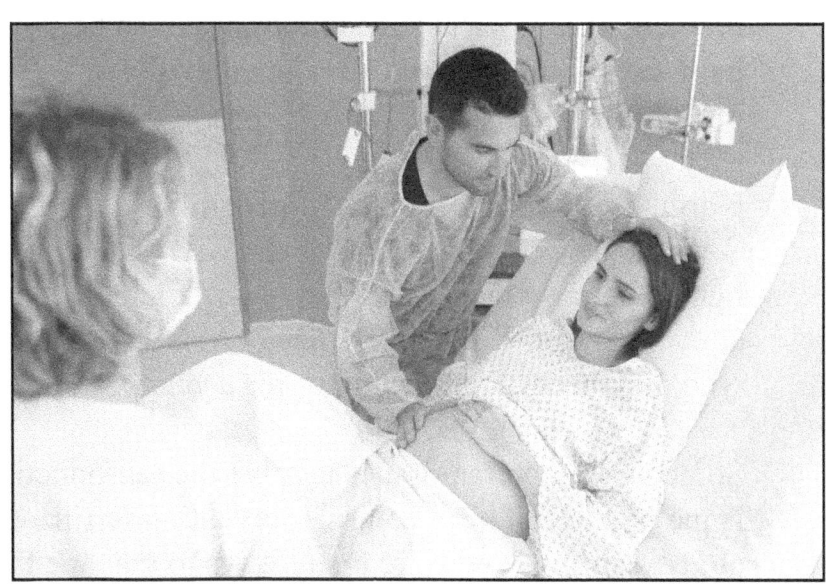

Giving birth in
a hospital maternity ward

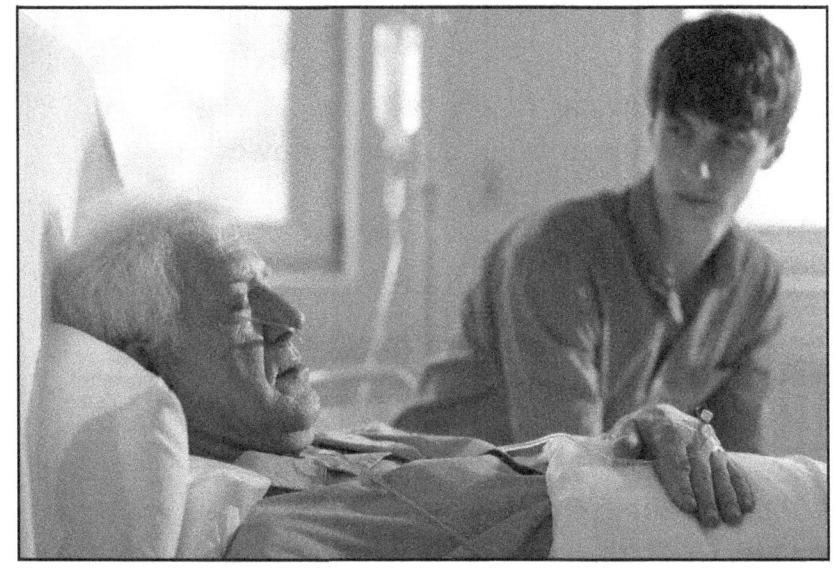

An elderly hospice
patient sleeping

Key Words

reproduction	sexual intercourse	fertilized	womb
pregnancy	labor	to deliver	to breastfeed
contraception	abortion	embryo/fetus	to circumcise
foreskin	penis	corpse	to cremate

READ

Birth and death are the most important dates in a human life, beginning and ending. Birth, however, is not the real beginning. In fact, it is the last moment of biological **reproduction**, which begins when man and woman have **sexual intercourse**. An egg is **fertilized** by sperm, and life begins in the **womb**.

Normally, after nine months of **pregnancy**, the woman goes into **labor**. With the help of a physician or midwife, she **delivers** a baby. A new human being comes from the body of a female human being. It is an amazing event. The helpless newborn is still dependent on its mother, who may **breastfeed** the infant for a year or more.*

Some very important issues involve the reproductive system. First is the practice of birth control, preventing fertilization, also called **contraception**. There are many ways to manage the sex act and prevent conception and eventual birth. The second issue involves **abortion**, which is removing the fertilized **embryo** or **fetus**** that will become a baby.

For the male child another important day can be the day he is **circumcised,** when the **foreskin** is removed from the **penis**. However, many parents choose not to have their child circumcised.

Death, the end, another great mystery, comes to all life. It can be sudden or slow, accidental or natural. The **corpse** may be **cremated** or buried. Usually there is a funeral or memorial service. *(232)*

* In some parts of the world today, some mothers do not nurse/breastfeed their babies. They bottlefeed them with their own milk or a formula similar to milk.

** The embryo becomes a fetus after eight weeks.

EXERCISES
(answers on page 65)

A. Match the two parts of the sentence.

1. Pregnancy lasts _____   A. soon after birth.
2. A midwife may help _____   B. cremated or buried.
3. An egg is fertilized _____   C. prevents fertilization.
4. She labored _____   D. on average nine months.
5. Contraception _____   E. also called nursing.
6. An embryo ____   F. becomes a fetus.
7. Circumcision may be done _____ G. result in fertilization.
8. The corpse will be _____   H. with the delivery.
9. Sexual intercourse can _____   I. for two hours.
10. Abortion is _____   J. illegal in some countries.
11. She carried the baby _____   K. by a sperm.
12. Breastfeeding is _____   L. in her womb.

B. Fill in the blanks.

1. All life _____ itself.
2. A baby forms in the _____.
3. A _____ woman is "carrying" a baby.
4. A sperm _____ an egg.
5. The woman may be in _____ for several hours.
6. _____ is also called breastfeeding.
7. The foreskin is removed from the _____.
8. Not having _____ is one form of contraception.
9. _____ involves removing the fetus before birth.
10. Do you want to be _____ or buried.

THINK ABOUT IT

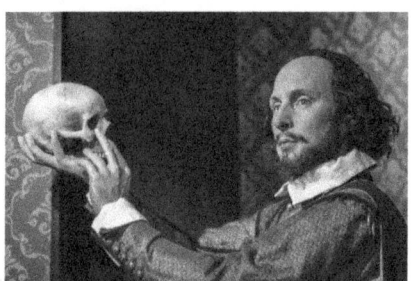

(**The Seven Ages of Man**, *from the play,* **As You Like It**, *is one of William Shakespeare's most famous speeches. Listen to and read the poem.*

Many of the words are no longer in common usage. On the right side of the page, make a list of the words you don't understand. Then search for the meaning.)

The Seven Ages of Man

All the world's a stage,
And all the men and women merely players;
They have their exits and their entrances,
And one man in his time plays many parts,
His acts being seven ages. At first the infant,
Mewling and puking in the nurse's arms.
Then, the whining school-boy with his satchel
And shining morning face, creeping like snail
Unwillingly to school. And then the lover,
Sighing like furnace, with a woeful ballad
Made to his mistress' eyebrow. Then, a soldier,
Full of strange oaths, and bearded like the pard,
Jealous in honour, sudden, and quick in quarrel,
Seeking the bubble reputation
Even in the cannon's mouth. And then, the justice,
In fair round belly, with good capon lined,
With eyes severe, and beard of formal cut,
Full of wise saws, and modern instances,
And so he plays his part. The sixth age shifts
Into the lean and slippered pantaloon,
With spectacles on nose and pouch on side,
His youthful hose, well saved, a world too wide
For his shrunk shank, and his big manly voice,
Turning again toward childish treble, pipes
And whistles in his sound. Last scene of all,
That ends this strange eventful history,
Is second childishness and mere oblivion,
Sans teeth, sans eyes, sans taste, sans everything.

(As You Like It, Act 2 Scene 7)

Health Answers

UNIT 1 Page 3
THE BODY

A. **Match**
1 – C
2 – I
3 – J
4 – H
5 – G
6 – A
7 – D
8 – E
9 – B
10 – K
11 – F

B. **Fill in**
1 – back
2 – hair
3 – chest, breasts
4 – hands
5 – legs
6 – male, female
7– male, female
8 – fingers, toes

UNIT 2 Page 7
THE SKELETON

A. **Match**
1 – E
2 – G
3 – H
4 – A
5 – B
6 – C
7 – I
8 – D
9 – F

B. **Fill in**
1 – skull
2 – jaw
3 – wrist
4 – elbow
5 – pelvis
6 – ankle, shin
7 – neck
8 – knee

UNIT 3 Page 11
THE FACE

A. **Match**
1 – E
2 – H
3 – J
4 – A
5 – B
6 – I
7 – C
8 – D
9 – G
10 – F

B. **Fill in**
1 – eyes
2 – chin
3 – mouth
4 – lips
5 – brown
6 – eyelids
7 – Eyelashes
8 – forehead
9 – cheeks
10 – smell, taste

UNIT 4 Page 15
EYES AND EARS

A. **Match**
   1 – E
   2 – I
   3 – F
   4 – C
   5 – G
   6 – A
   7 – K
   8 – J
   9 – B
  10 – H
  11 – D

B. **Fill in**
   1 – dizzy
   2 – inner ear
   3 – vision/eyesight
   4 – ringing
   5 – tinnitus
   6 – blurry
   7 – mute
   8 – sore
   9 – infection, throat/tonsils
  10 – vision

UNIT 5 Page 19
THE DIGESTIVE TRACT

A. **Match**
   1 – F
   2 – D
   3 – G
   4 – H
   5 – C
   6 – A
   7 – I
   8 – B
   9 – E

B. **Fill in**
   1 – chew(ed), swallow(ed)
   2 – esophagus
   3 – Indigestion
   4 – intestine(s)
   5 – Appendicitis
   6 – anus
   7 – diarrhea, constipated
   8 – rectum, colon

UNIT 6 Page 23
**THE HEART, LUNGS
AND OTHER ORGANS**

A. **Match**
   1 – C
   2 – E
   3 – D
   4 – I
   5 – A
   6 – F
   7 – H
   8 – G
   9 – B

B. **Fill in**
   1 – breath
   2 – liver/kidneys
   3 – Veins, arteries, cells
   4 – inhale, oxygen, lungs
   5 – exhale
   6 – absorbs
   7 – enzymes
   8 – bladder, urine
   9 – cells
  10 – pump

UNIT 7 Page 27
ILLNESS, ALLERGY, AND DISEASE

A. **Match**
1 – H
2 – F
3 – I
4 – D
5 – E
6 – B
7 – C
8 – A
9 – G

B. **Fill in**
1 – Tuberculosis
2 – cancer
3 – fracture
4 – pandemic
5 – twist(ed), ankle
6 – rash
7 – cough, sneeze
8 – flu
9 – pneumonia/tuberculosis
10 – symptom

UNIT 8 Page 31
THE DOCTOR'S OFFICE

A. **Match**
1 – H
2 – G
3 – I
4 – A
5 – F
6 – E
7 – D
8 – B
9 – C

B. **Fill in**
1 – healthcare
2 – waiting room, examination room
3 – appointment, receptionist
4 – pressure
5 – over
6 – urgent, emergency
7 – prescribe
8 – specialist

UNIT 9 Page 35
AT THE DENTIST

A. **Match**
1 – F
2 – G
3 – J
4 – A
5 – B
6 – H
7 – I
8 – D
9 – C
10 – K
11 – E

B. **Fill in**
1 – anesthetic
2 – brush, floss
3 – Braces
4 – Medication
5 – gums
6 – hygienist
7 – Pain, syringe
8 – infected, extracted
9 – root canal
10 – decayed/infected

UNIT 10 Page 39
THE HOSPITAL

A. **Match**
1 – K
2 – E
3 – G
4 – H
5 – J
6 – I
7 – F
8 – A
9 – D
10 – B
11 – C

B. **Fill in**
1 – delivery room
2 – operating
3 – outpatient
4 – admissions
5 – radiology
6 – anesthetic
7 – surgeon
8 – severe
9 – tumor
10 – ambulance
11 – scan
12 – intensive care

UNIT 11 Page 43
NUTRITION

A. **Match**
1 – I
2 – F
3 – J
4 – E
5 – A
6 – B
7 – C
8 – G
9 – H
10 – D

B. **Fill in**
1 – nutritionist, diet
2 – calories
3 – carbohydrates
4 – starch
5 – nutritious
6 – muscles
7 – obese
8 – quantity

UNIT 12 Page 47
EXERCISE

A. **Match**
1 – K
2 – I
3 – F
4 – H
5 – J
6 – A
7 – D
8 – B
9 – C
10 – G
11 – E

B. **Fill in**
1 – Aerobic, anaerobic
2 – weight
3 – aerobic
4 – muscles
5 – risk
6 – fitness, gym
7 – weight
8 – routine

MENTAL HEALTH

A. **Match**
  1 – D
  2 – G
  3 – I
  4 – C
  5 – H
  6 – B
  7 – A
  8 – E
  9 – F

B. **Fill in**
  1 – suffers, addiction
  2 – disorder(s)
  3 – cope, reality/stress
  4 – Substance/Drug
  5 – productive
  6 – quit
  7 – chronic
  8 – alcoholic
  9 – psychosis
  10 – prevention

PUBLIC HEALTH

A. **Match**
  1 – F
  2 – J
  3 – H
  4 – A
  5 – I
  6 – B
  7 – C
  8 – K
  9 – E
  10 – G
  11 – D

B. **Fill in**
  1 – Vaccinations
  2 – contagious/ infectious
  3 – infectious/ contagious
  4 – Maintaining
  5 – Prevention
  6 – crisis
  7 – protected
  8 – personal protective
  9 – virus

BIRTH AND DEATH

A. **Match**
  1 – D
  2 – H
  3 – K
  4 – I
  5 – C
  6 – F
  7 – A
  8 – B
  9 – G
  10 – J
  11 – L
  12 – E

B. **Fill in**
  1 – reproduces
  2 – womb
  3 – pregnant
  4 – fertilizes
  5 – labor
  6 – Nursing
  7 – penis
  8 – sexual intercourse
  9 – Abortion
  10 – cremated

Key Word List

This list locates the first occurrence of each lexical item. The number indicates the unit.

abortion 15	blurry 4	constipation 5	elbow 2
to absorb 6	braces 9	contagious 14	embryo 15
addiction 13	breast 1	to contain 14	emergency 8
admissions 10	to breastfeed 15	contraception 15	enzymes 6
aerobic 12	to breathe 6	to cope 13	epidemic 7
alcoholism 13	to brush 9	corpse 15	esophagus 5
ambulance 10	calorie 11	to/a cough 7	examination room 8
anaerobic 12	cancer 7	to cremate 15	to exhale 6
to anesthetize 10	carbohydrate 11	crisis 14	to extract 9
ankle 2	cardiovascular 12	crown 9	eye 3
anus 5	cavity 9	CT scan 10	eyebrow 3
appendix 5	cells 6	deaf 4	eyelash 3
appointment 8	cheek 3	to decay 9	eyelid 3
arm 1	chest 1	to deliver 15	female 1
arteries 6	to chew 5	delivery room 10	fertilized 15
balance 4	chin 3	diabetes 6	fetus 15
balanced diet 11	chronic 13	diarrhea 5	fiber 11
benefits 12	to circumcise 15	disorder 13	filling 9
bladder 6	clinic 8	dizziness 4	filter 6
blind 4	collective 14	to drill 9	finger 1
blood pressure 8	colon 5	earache 4	fitness 12

 Key Word List

to floss 9

foot 1

forehead 3

foreskin 15

to/a fracture 7

grains 11

gum 9

gym 12

hair 1

hand 1

head 1

healthcare
   provider 8

heart attack 7

height 8

herd immunity 14

hip 2

hygienist 9

indigestion 5

infected 4

infectious 14

to inhale 6

to inject 9

inner ear 4

intensive 12

intensive care unit
   (ICU) 10

intestine 5

jaw 2

jogging 12

knee 2

labor 15

lab(oratory) 10

leg 1

lip 3

liver 6

to maintain 14

male 1

maternity 10

medication 9

mineral 11

mouth 3

MRI 10

muscles 11

mute 4

neck 2

needle 9

normal 13

nose 3

nutrient 11

nutritionist 11

obese 11

operating room
   (OR) 10

orthodontist 9

outpatient 10

pancreas 6

pandemic 7

to peak 14

pelvis 2

penis 15

permanent 9

pharmaceutical 14

pneumonia 7

pregnancy 15

to prescribe 8

preventable 13

primary care 8

processed 11

productively 13

protective 14

protein 11

psychotic 13

to pump 6

quantity 11

to quit 13

radiology 10

rash 7

receptionist 8

rectum 5

reproduction 15

ringing ears 4

risk 12

root canal 9

routine 12

runny 7

severe 10

sexual
   intercourse 15

shin 2

shoulder 2

skull 2

to smell 3	substance abuse 13	toe 1	virus 14
to sneeze 7	to suffer 13	tonsils 4	vision 4
sore throat 4	surgery 10	tuberculosis 7	vitamin 11
specialist 8	to swallow 5	tumor 10	waiting room 8
spine 2	symptoms 7	to twist 7	weight 8
sprain 7	syringe 9	urgent 8	weightlifting 12
spread 14	to taste 3	urine 6	weight loss 12
starch 11	thigh 2	vaccine 14	womb 15
stomach 1	throat 5	veins 6	wrist 2
stress 13	tinnitus 4	vertebrae 2	x-ray 10